Book of Sayings

PETA ZAFIR

Book of Sayings

Book 6

©2022 Peta Zafir

All rights reserved.

No part of this book may be reproduced in any form or by any electronic or mechanical means, including information storage and retrieval systems, without written permission from the author, except in the case of a reviewer, who may quote brief passages embodied in critical articles or in a review.

Trademarked names appear throughout this book. Rather than use a trademark symbol with every occurrence of a trademarked name, names are used in an editorial fashion, with no intention of infringement of the respective owner's trademark.

The information in this book is distributed on an "as is" basis, without warranty. Although every precaution has been taken in the preparation of this work, neither the author nor the publisher shall have any liability to any person or entity with respect to any loss or damage caused or alleged to be caused directly or indirectly by the information contained in this book.

Peta Zafir Publishing
www.petazafir.com

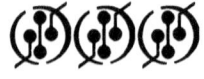

ISBN 978-0-6452140-8-6

Peta Zafir Publishing
www.petazafir.com
Peta Zafir You Tube Channel

BOOKS BY PETA ZAFIR
Health in Poetry Book 1
Health in Poetry Book 2
Book of Sayings Book 1
Book of Sayings Book 2
Book of Sayings Book 3
Book of Sayings Book 4
Book of Sayings Book 5
Book of Sayings Book 6
Scenar For Beginners
Book of Sayings Book 1 in Italian

All books are available in print and eBook format from:
www.petazafir.com/books

Dedication

To all those people clearing away their past experiences, working to create serenity, happiness and peace in the present, all leading to a full and wonderful future.

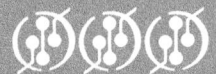

Book of Sayings   Book 6

Access your Past

Work on it

Make alterations

Accept it then Move Forward

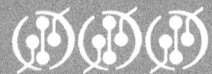

Book of Sayings   Book 6

Your Past explains your Influences
However You create who YOU will Be

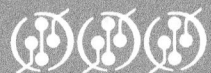

Book of Sayings   Book 6

I perceive myself as I am
Strive for my ideal and
Realize my human limitations

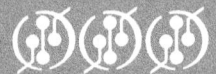

Book of Sayings   Book 6

Tyranny only has a voice when we allow it to speak

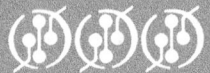

Book of Sayings   Book 6

Remember the Past

Look forward to the Future

Live in the Present

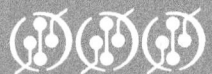

Book of Sayings   Book 6

Don't Change yourself to
Fit Another's requirements

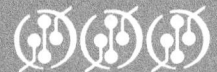

Book of Sayings   Book 6

There are many changeovers in Life
Feel them, understand the change
Work out what you want and
How you're going to Progress

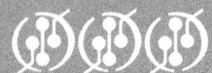

Book of Sayings   Book 6

There is a Time for all Things
And the Loss of all Things

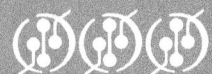

Book of Sayings   Book 6

Do not pursue those things
that are detrimental to you

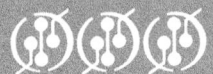

Book of Sayings   Book 6

Some Feelings are to be Fixed and Mended, and

Some Feelings just are

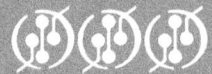

Book of Sayings   Book 6

Not every Emotion can be changed
Feel it, Work through it, and
Then travel forwards

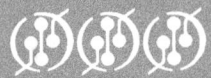

Book of Sayings   Book 6

Past experiences can never be recaptured

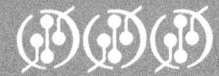

Book of Sayings   Book 6

Don't allow yourself
to waste the time you have

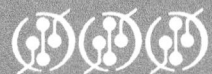

Book of Sayings   Book 6

Youth does not give you Time

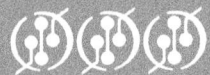

Book of Sayings Book 6

Value your life
Cherish your Family
Make your priorities

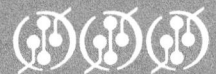

Book of Sayings   Book 6

Every day you need to work on and create

The Life you Want

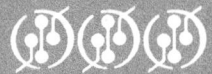

Book of Sayings   Book 6

Life offers us Time
To grow into the person
You were born to be

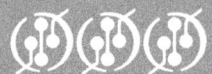

Book of Sayings   Book 6

Live in the Essence of Simplicity

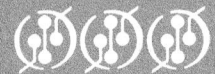

Book of Sayings   Book 6

You have a right to create a boundary
You have a right to speak you truth
Speak slowly and softly and walk forward

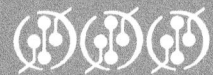

Book of Sayings   Book 6

Don't Live looking Back

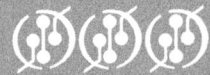

Book of Sayings   Book 6

Never judge yourself on past events
Review them, understand them
Change your behaviour
And act differently

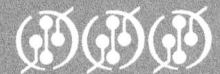

Book of Sayings   Book 6

Best choices every day with
the Best Health you have at the time

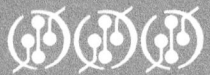

Book of Sayings   Book 6

Regrow and Rebuild

Or Don't

Your Choice

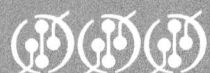

Book of Sayings   Book 6

Don't Let your Past
Compound your Future

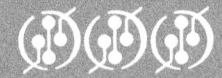

Book of Sayings   Book 6

How much do you Value
Having a Life that's worth having

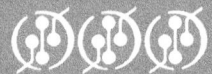

Book of Sayings   Book 6

Secrets are Sick
So, Speak your truth
Secrets are Sick

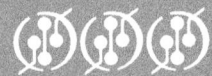

Book of Sayings   Book 6

You can overcome anything

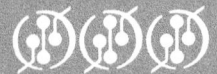

Book of Sayings   Book 6

Live your Life with
Innocence and Simplicity

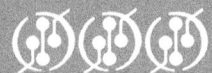

Book of Sayings   Book 6

Life's Experiences are a
Process of Learning

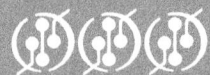

Book of Sayings   Book 6

Simplicity in Life gives us
Serenity, Peace and Connection

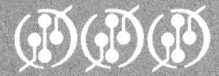

Book of Sayings   Book 6

Every small step
Brings you
Closer to your Goal

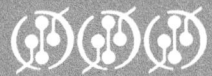

BOOK OF SAYINGS   BOOK 6

Clear the Past to
Create the Future

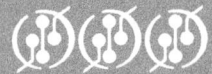

Book of Sayings   Book 6

Don't cloud your future
By dragging your Past behind

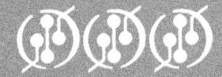

Book of Sayings   Book 6

If you take toxic people and events
To go into the next step of your life
Then you are allowing others
To influence your happiness and
The Journey you will have

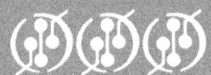

Book of Sayings   Book 6

Don't give others your Power

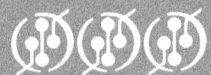

Book of Sayings   Book 6

Your reactions in Life
Result in your action or inactions
Choose your path

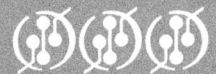

Don't be consumed by life

Value what you have and

Look forward to what you are wanting to achieve

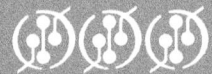

Book of Sayings   Book 6

Through hard work and saving
You appreciate what you acquire

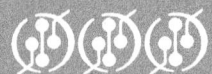

Book of Sayings   Book 6

Make your decisions using your
Mental, Emotional and Physical Maturity

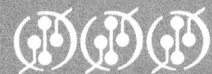

Book of Sayings   Book 6

Only spend what you have and
Only spend what you can afford to spend

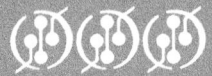

Appreciate and Respect others
Don't take anyone for granted
Life can change so quickly

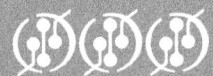

Book of Sayings   Book 6

You cannot bring someone into your future
If they don't want to come

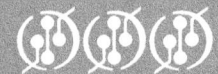

Book of Sayings   Book 6

If you want someone to act like a responsible adult then you need to treat them like a responsible adult

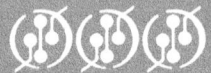

Book of Sayings   Book 6

Children need happy Parents
Not parents that stay together for the children

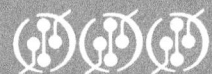

Book of Sayings   Book 6

Know what you want,
Communicate this
Work out the Balance and
Find the compromise

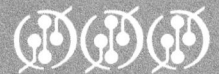

Book of Sayings   Book 6

Create the Life & relationship you want
Live your life, like you have only today

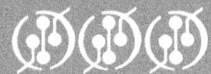

Book of Sayings   Book 6

If today you are missing something
Find out what it is
And stop and do it

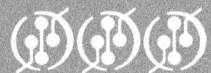

Book of Sayings   Book 6

Create more memories
And No more Regrets

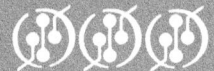

Book of Sayings   Book 6

You are never too young to learn and understand the concept of

Saving, earning and the value of Money

Peta Zafir Publishing
www.petazafir.com
Peta Zafir You Tube Channel

BOOKS BY PETA ZAFIR
Health in Poetry Book 1
Health in Poetry Book 2
Book of Sayings Book 1
Book of Sayings Book 2
Book of Sayings Book 3
Book of Sayings Book 4
Book of Sayings Book 5
Book of Sayings Book 6
Scenar For Beginners
Book of Sayings Book 1 in Italian

All books are available in print and eBook format from:
www.petazafir.com/books

www.ingramcontent.com/pod-product-compliance
Lightning Source LLC
Chambersburg PA
CBHW072338300426
44109CB00042B/1760